Beautiful Christmas Coloring Book

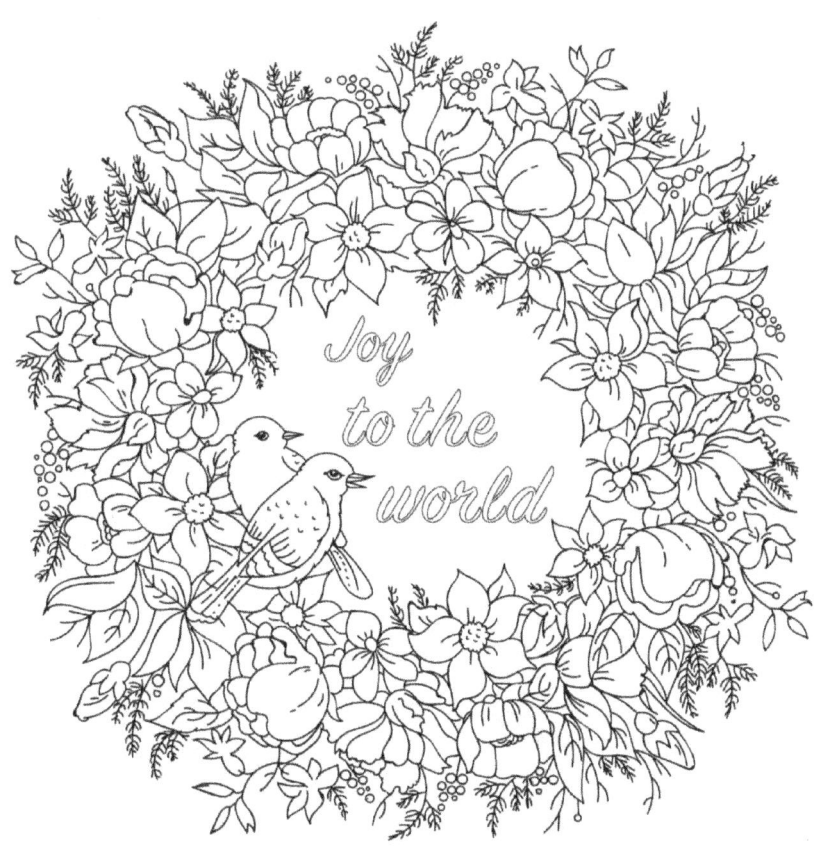

By Lucinda Crawford

Adult Coloring Book Series

This Coloring Book Belongs To

_____

Date _____

Table of Content

Image 1   Angel with Flute

Image 2   Joy

Image 3   Christmas Market Stand

Image 4   Christmas Tree with Doodle Background

Image 5   Elk Christmas Wreath

Image 6   Christmas Bells

Image 7   Christmas Market Mugs

Image 8   Festive Christmas Table Setting

Image 9   Gift Wrapping

Image 10   Joy-Love-Hope-Peace Tree

Image 11   Owl Ornament

Image 12   Joy to the World Wreath

Image 13   St. Nicolaus Boot

Image 14   Festive Home Entrance

Image 15   Nativity Scene

Image 16   Christmas Ball Ornaments

Image 17   Christmas Sweater with Hat and Mittens

Image 18   Stars

Image 19   Merry Christmas Door Wreath

Image 20   Fireplace Mantel with Elk

Image 21   Angel with Harp

Image 22   Christmas Cookies with Two Cups of Coffee

Image 23   Festive Advent Table Décor with Candles

Image 24   Christmas Tree

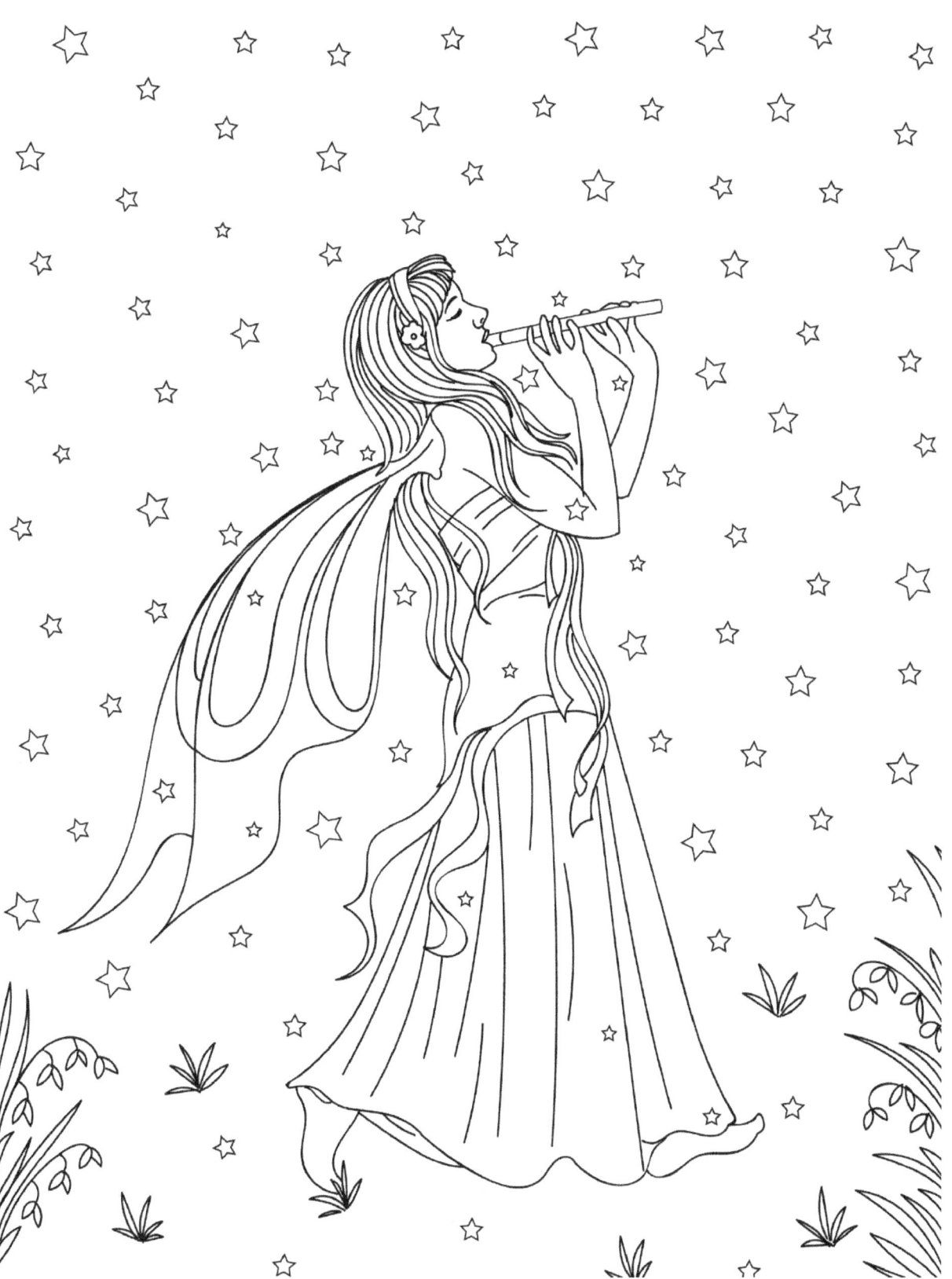

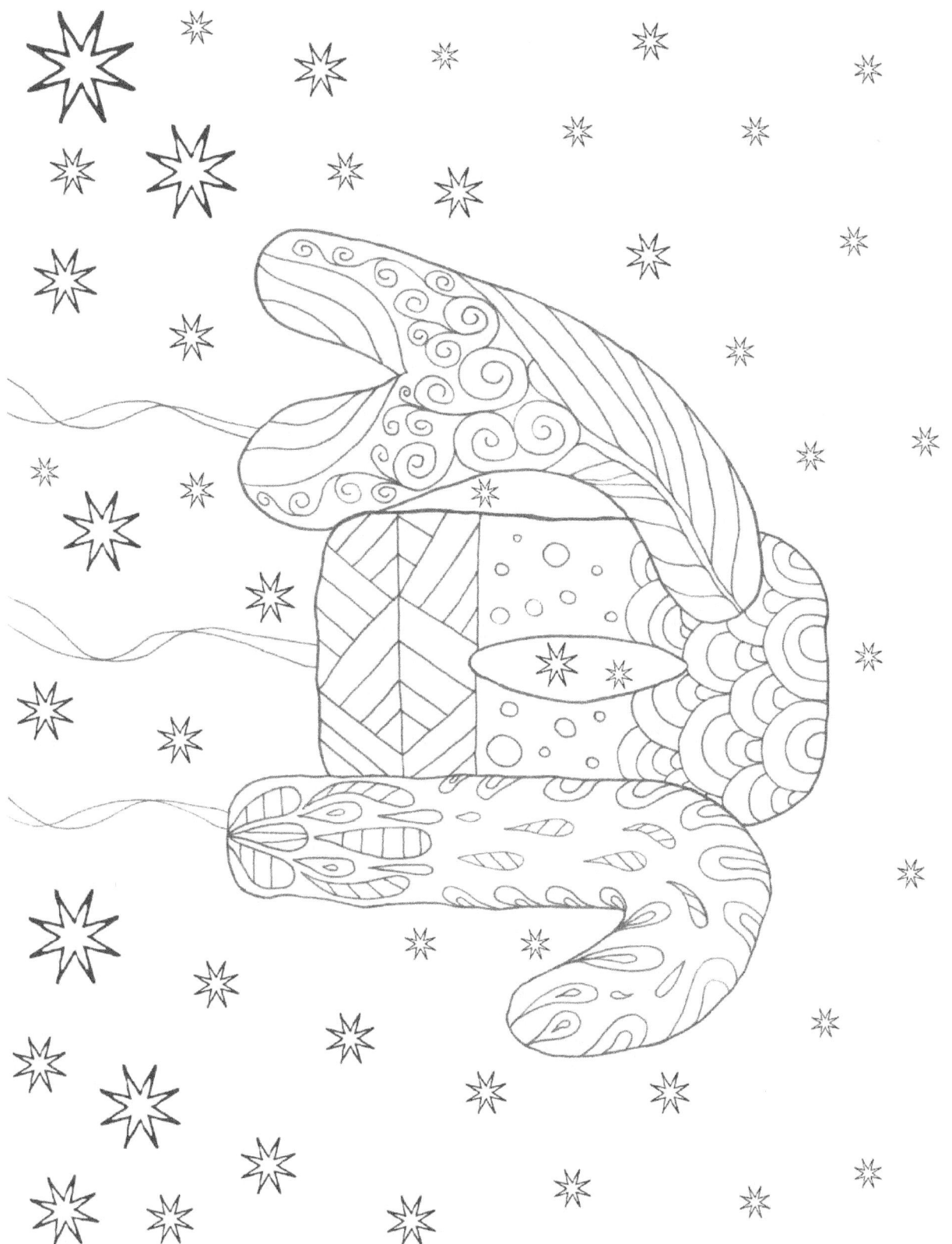

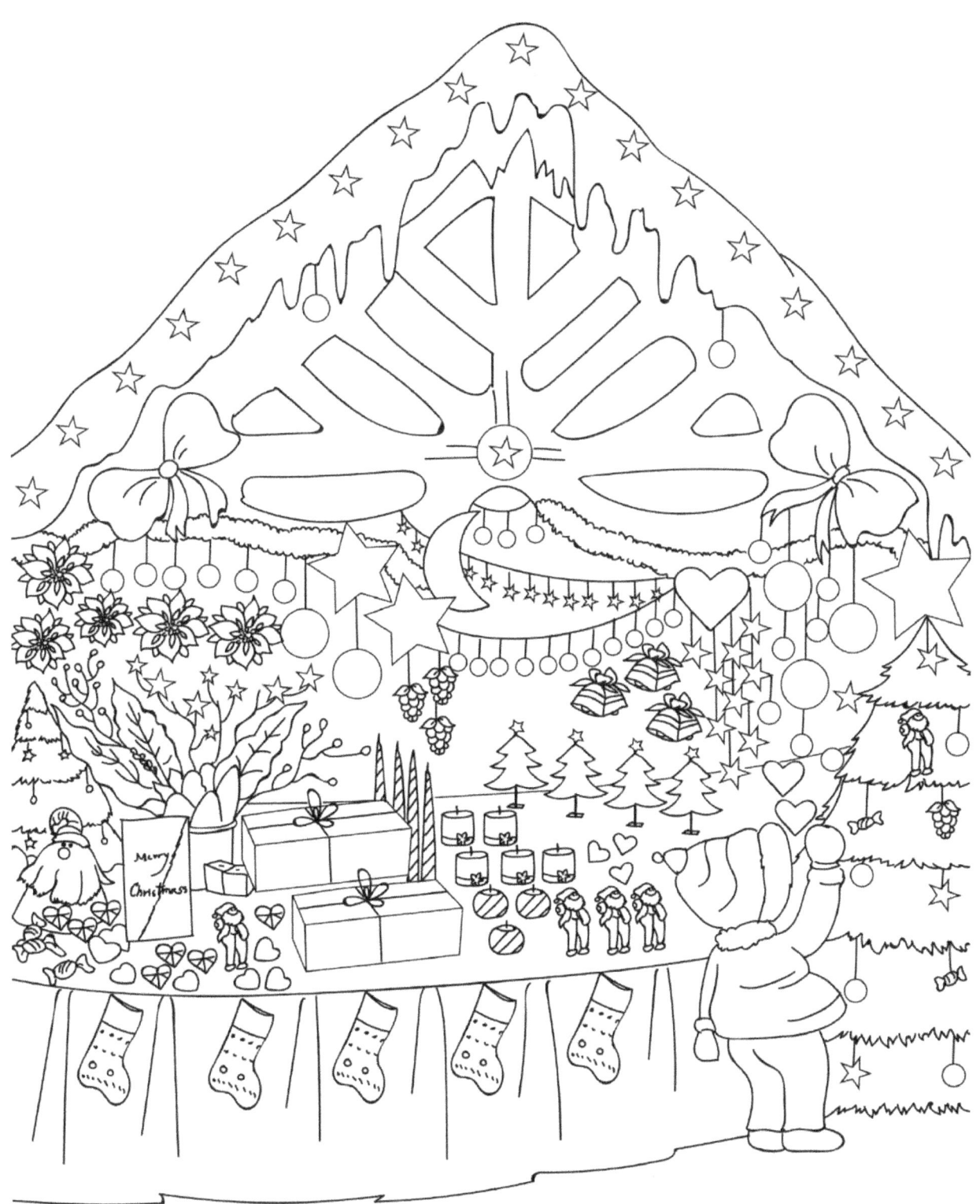

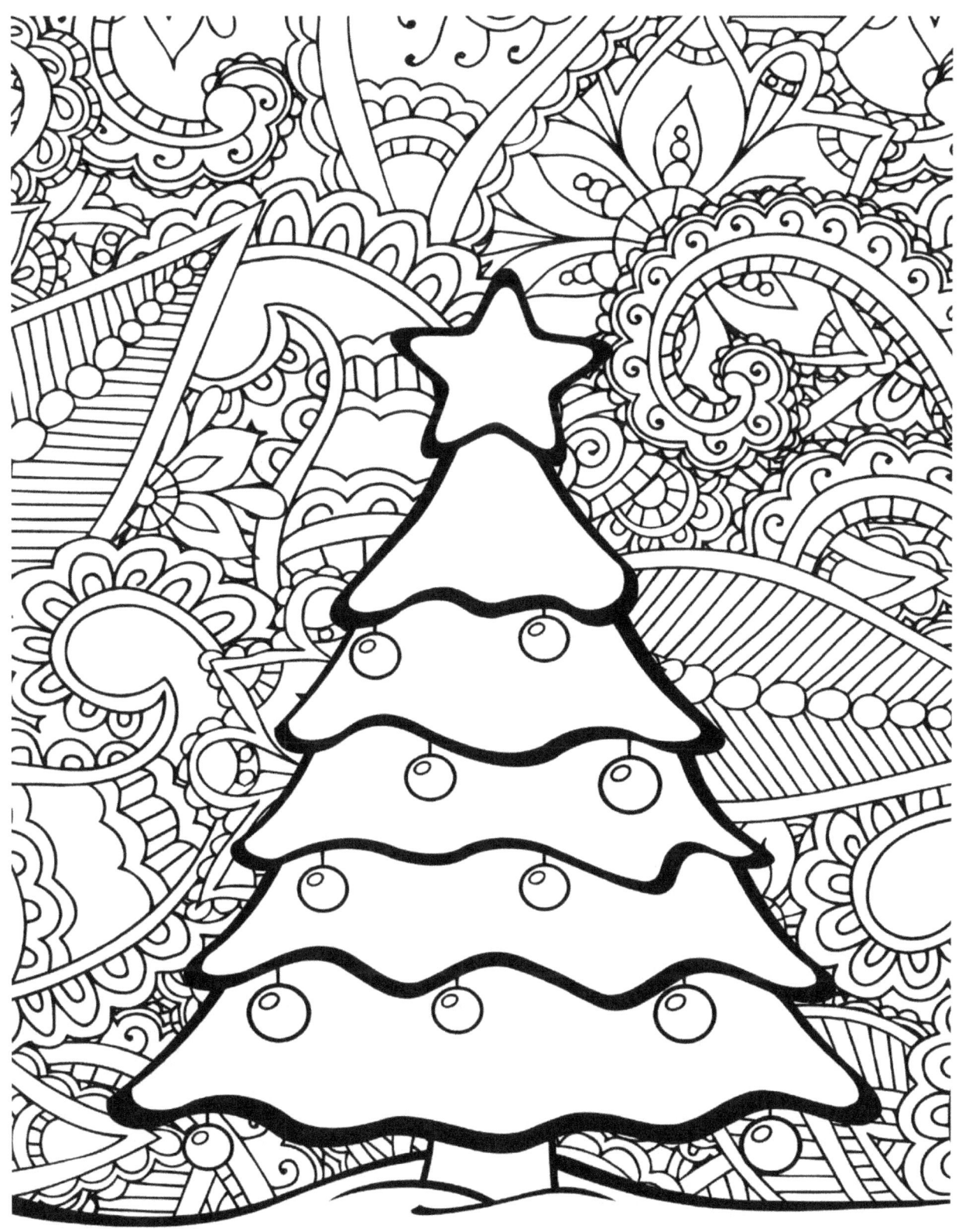

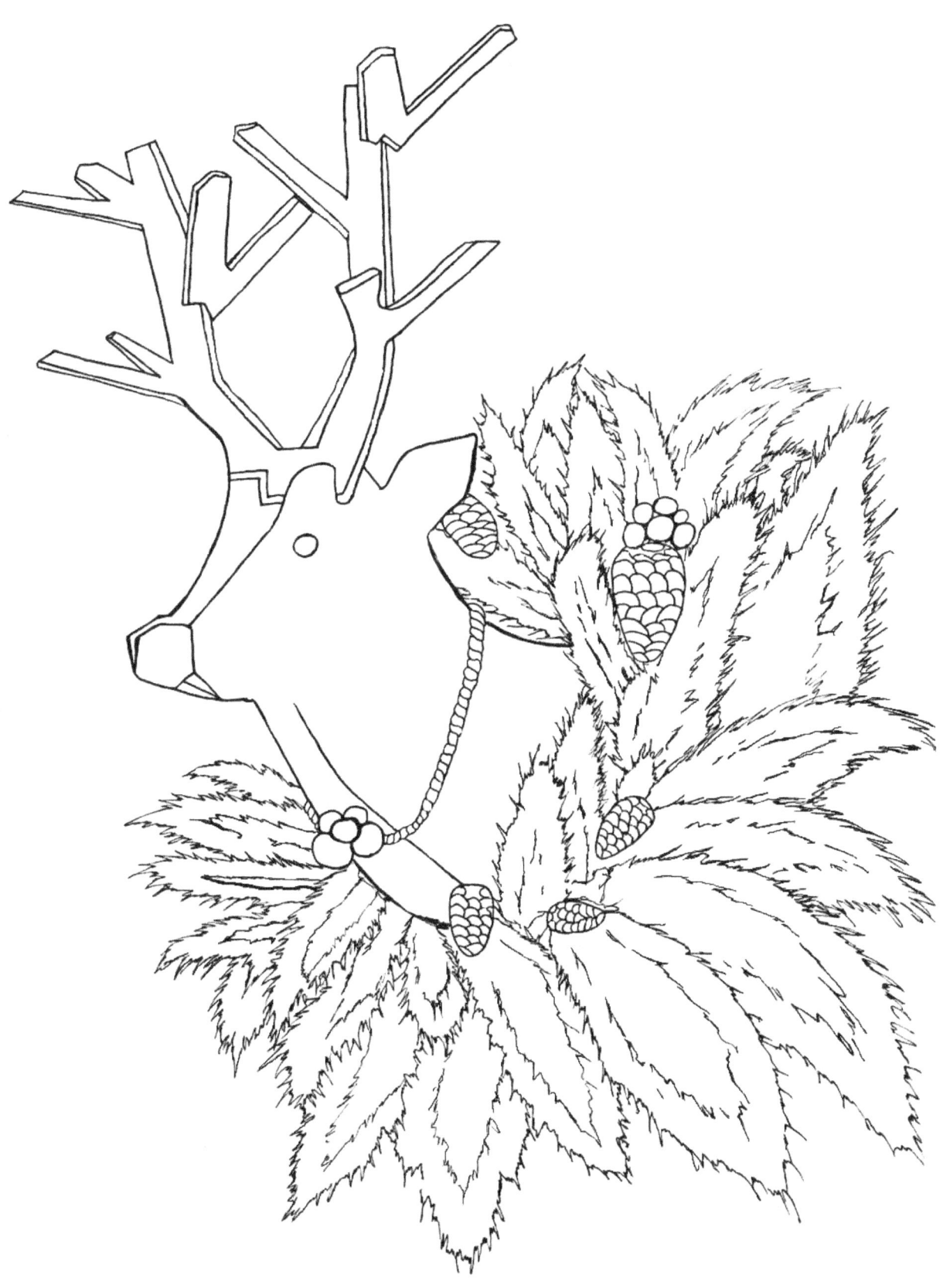

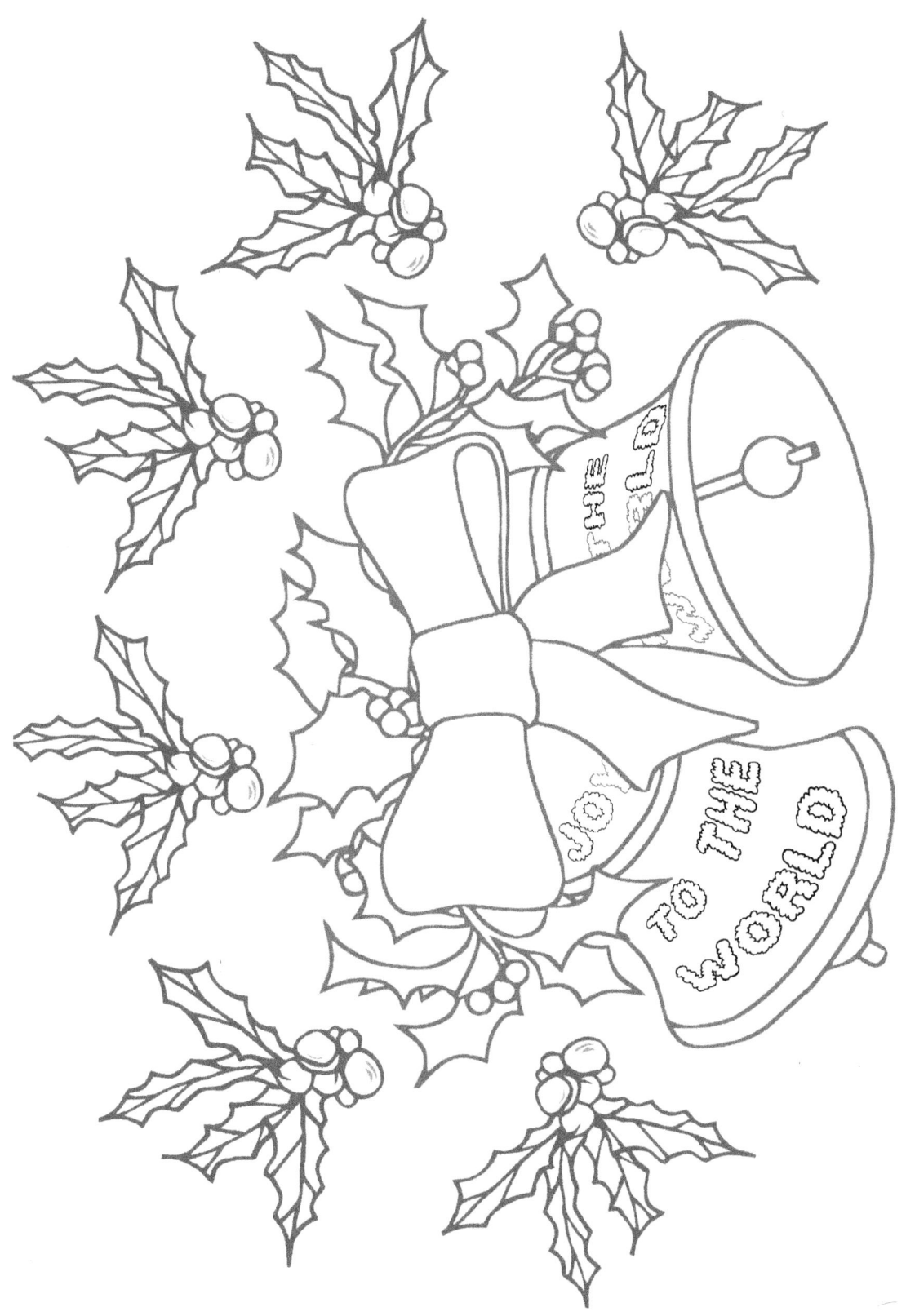

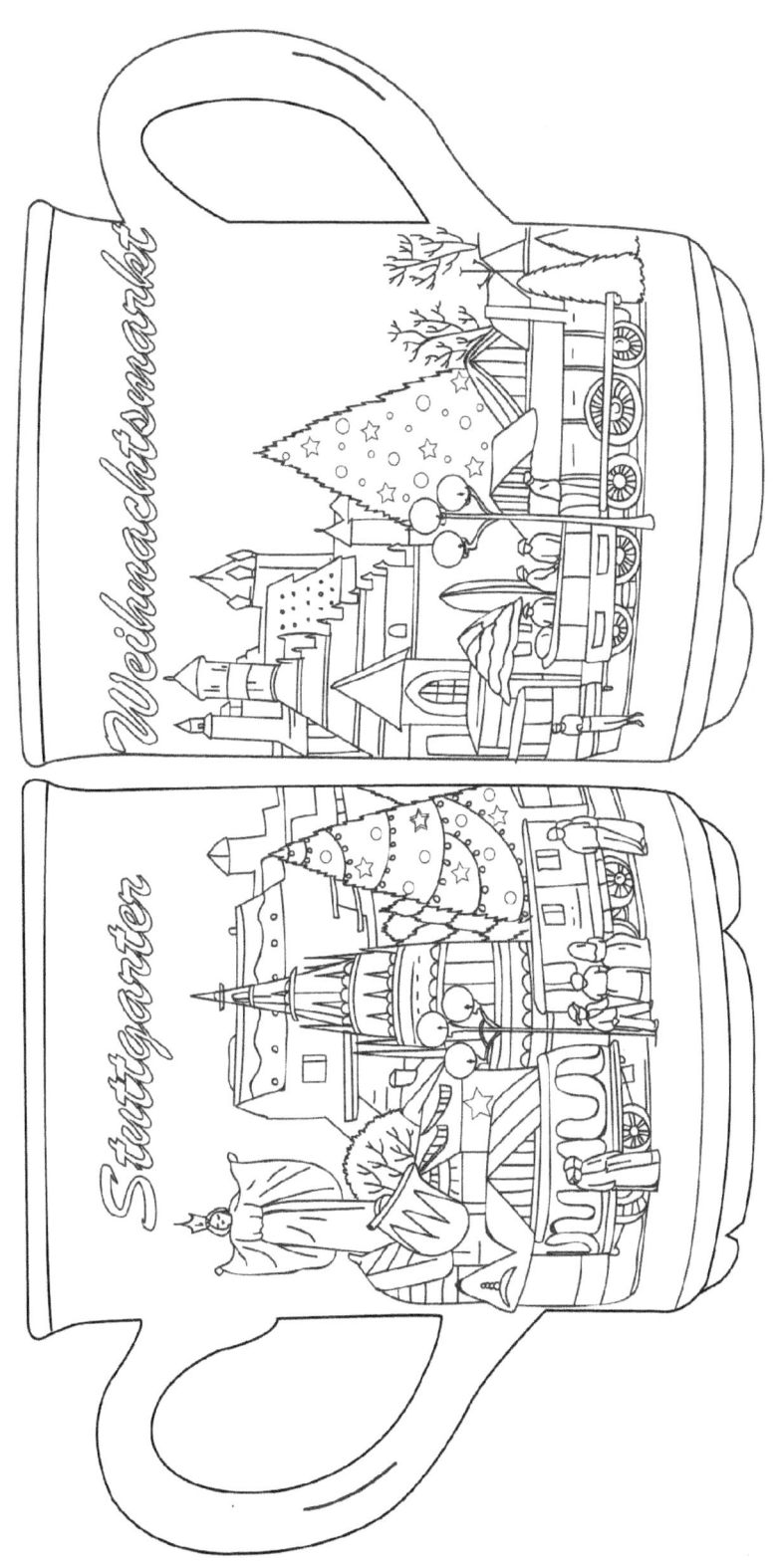

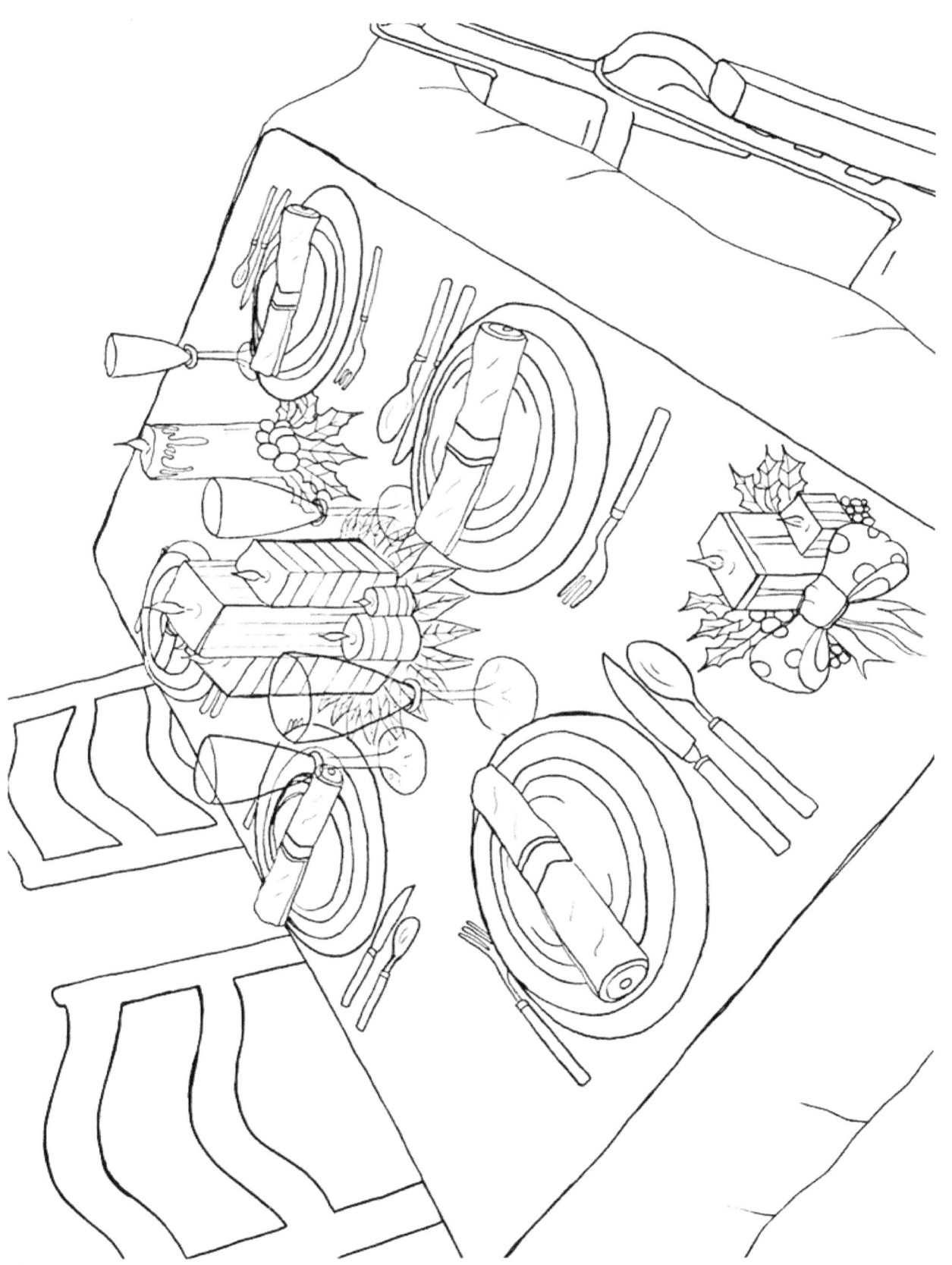

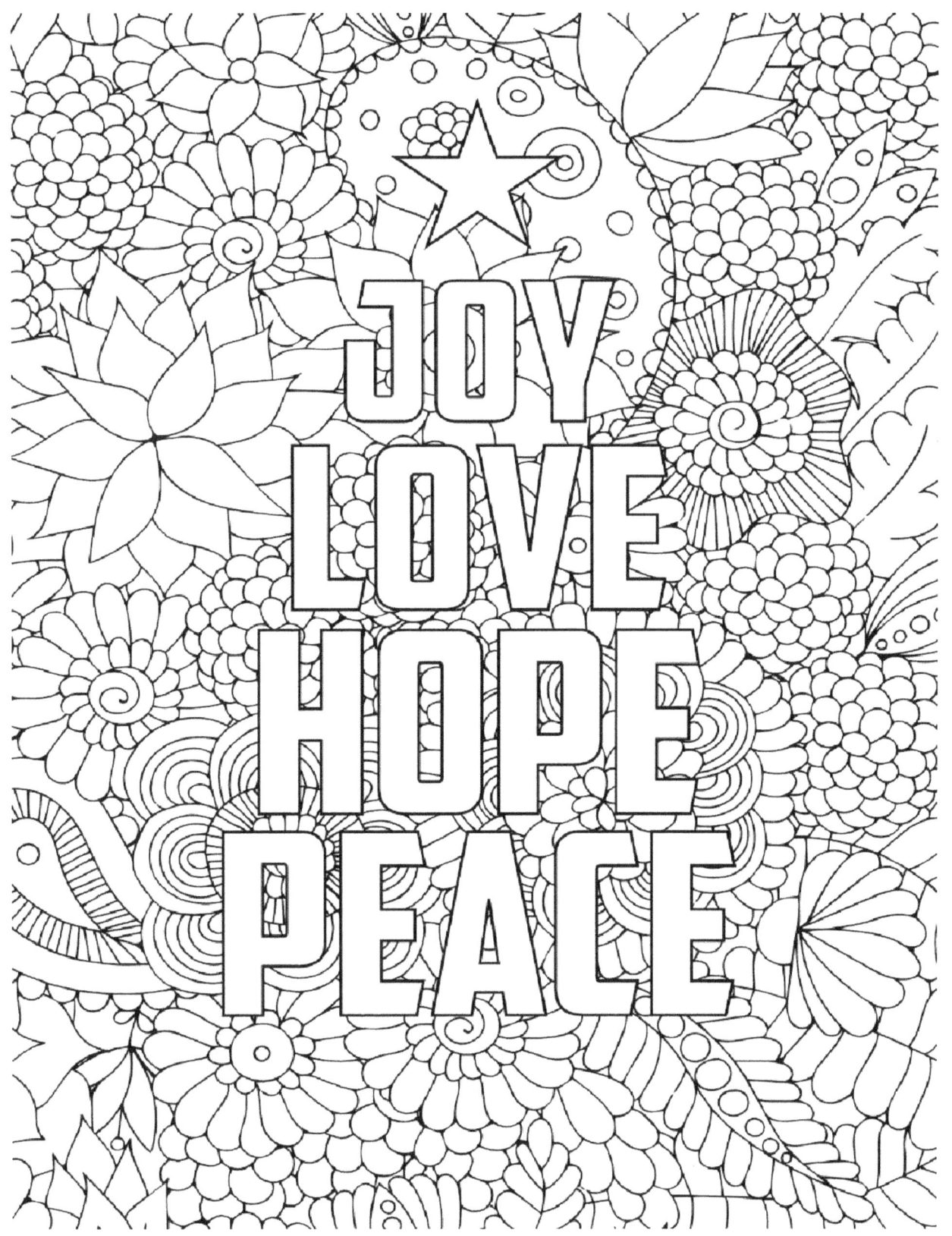

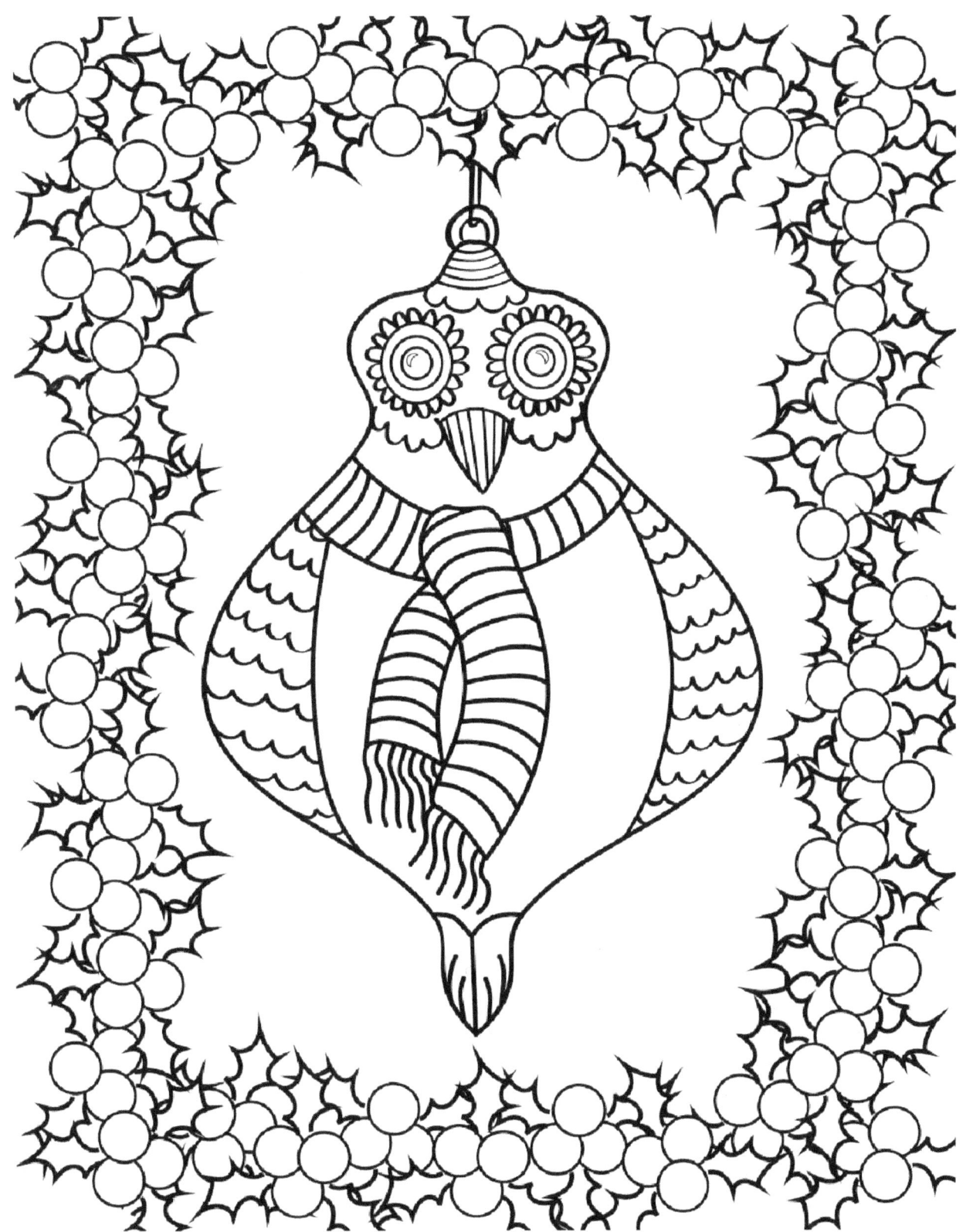

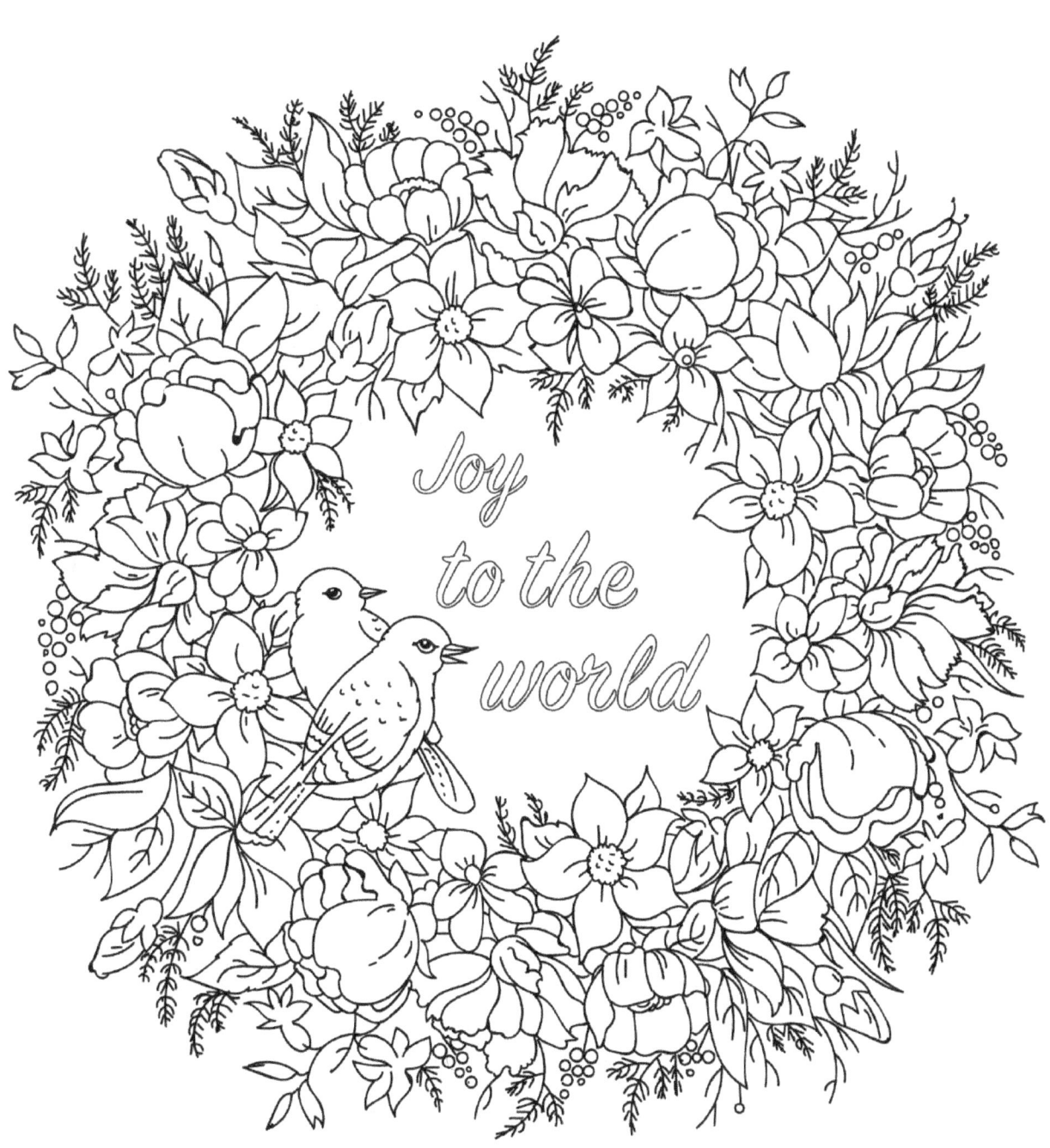

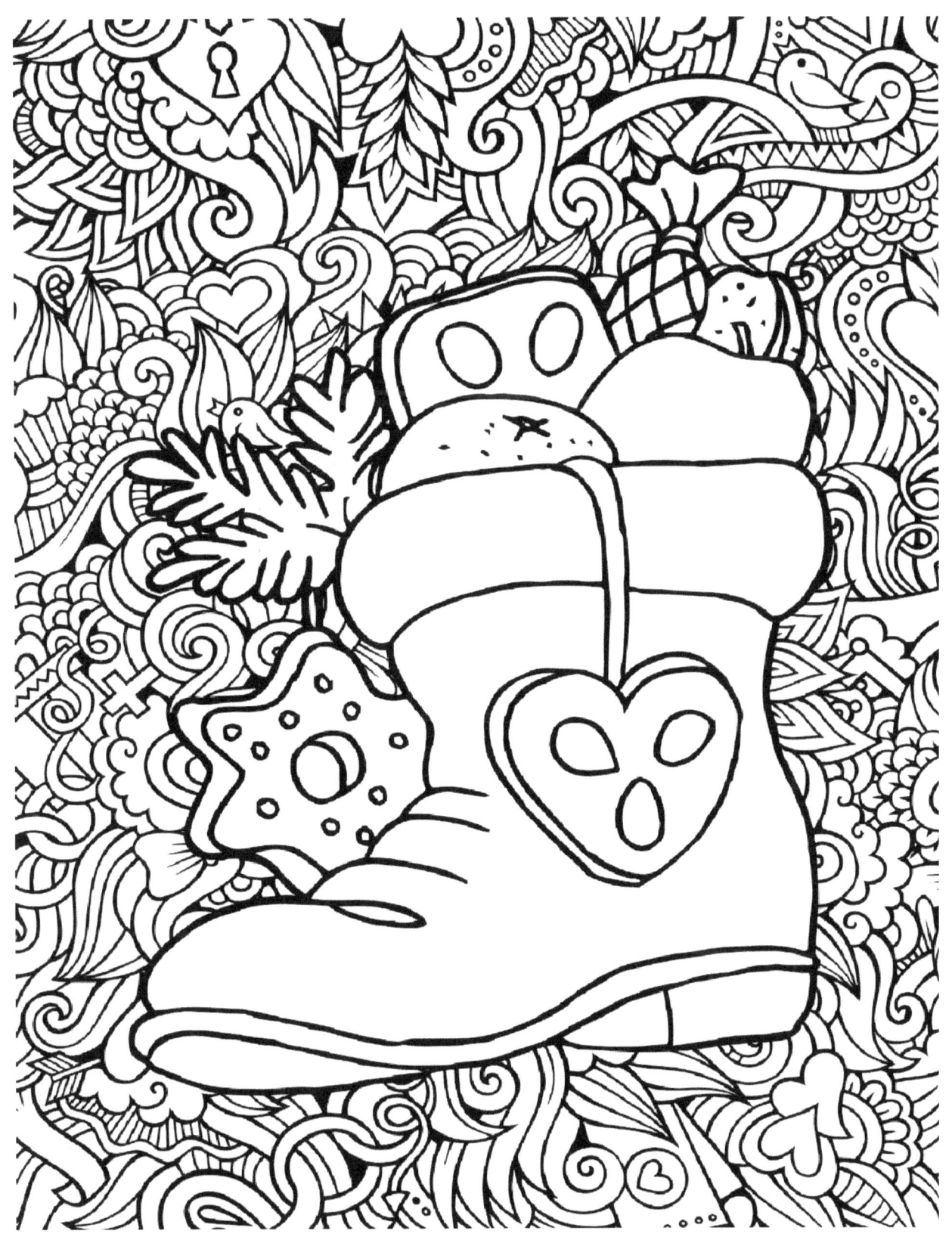

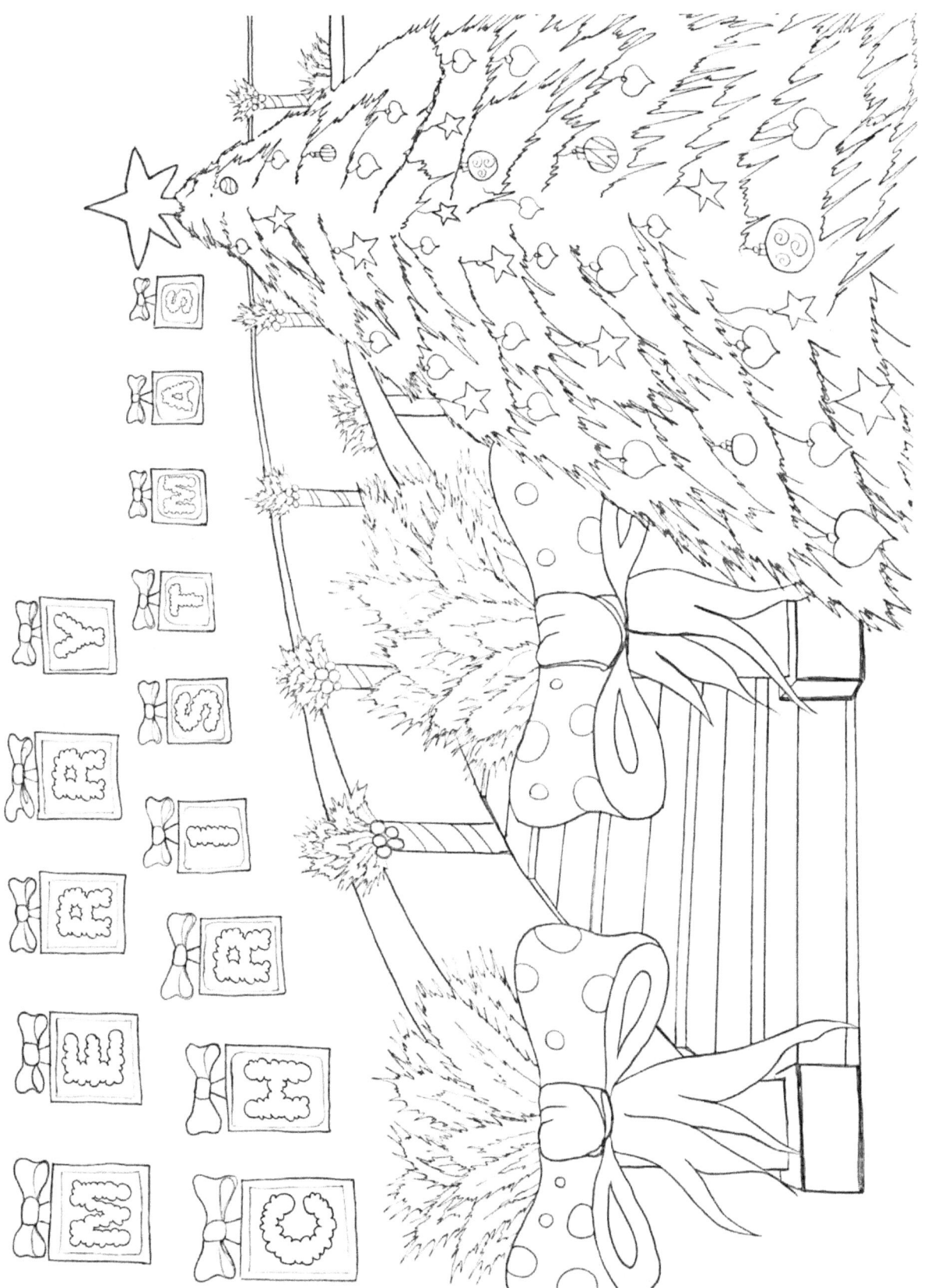

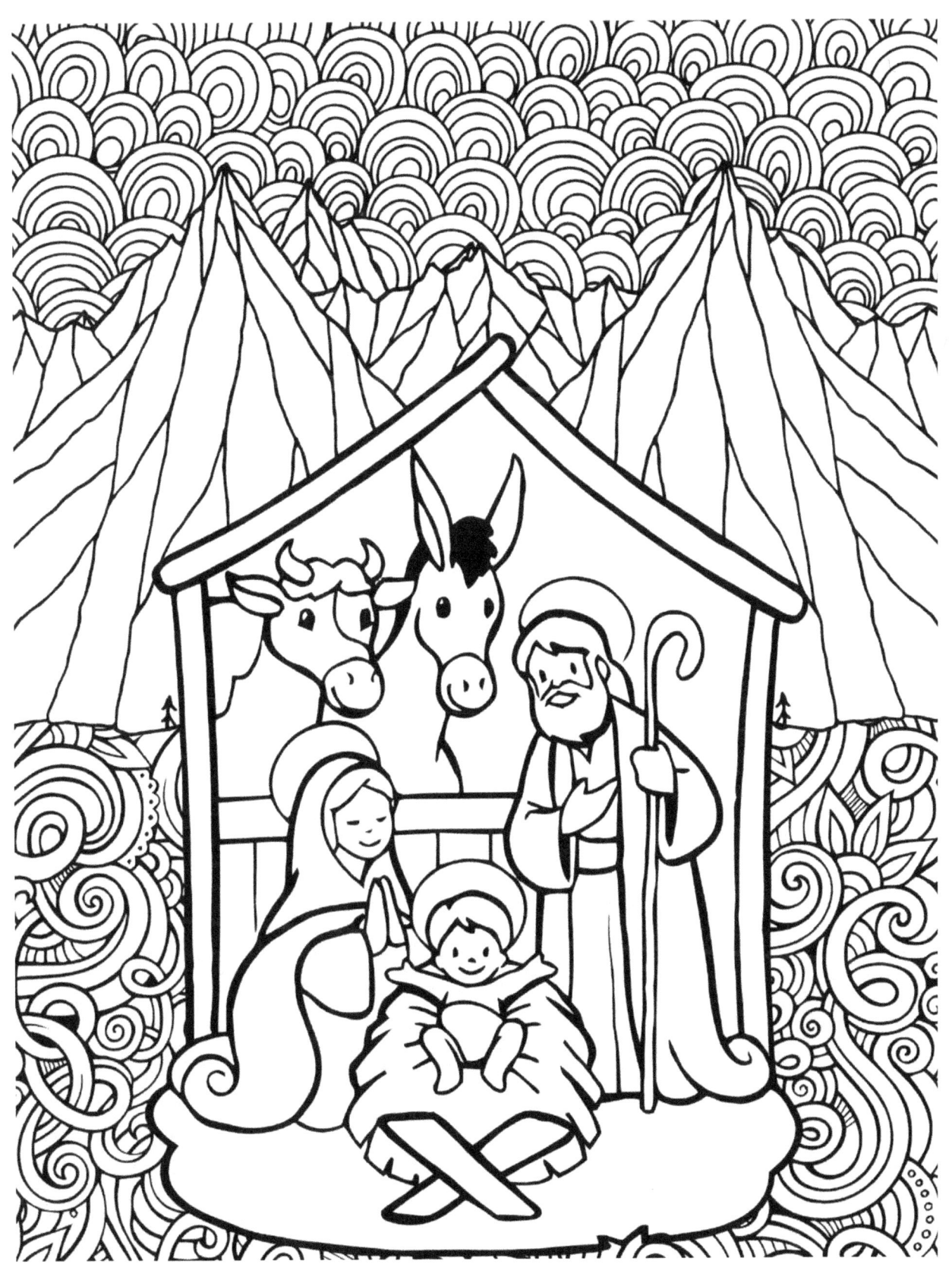

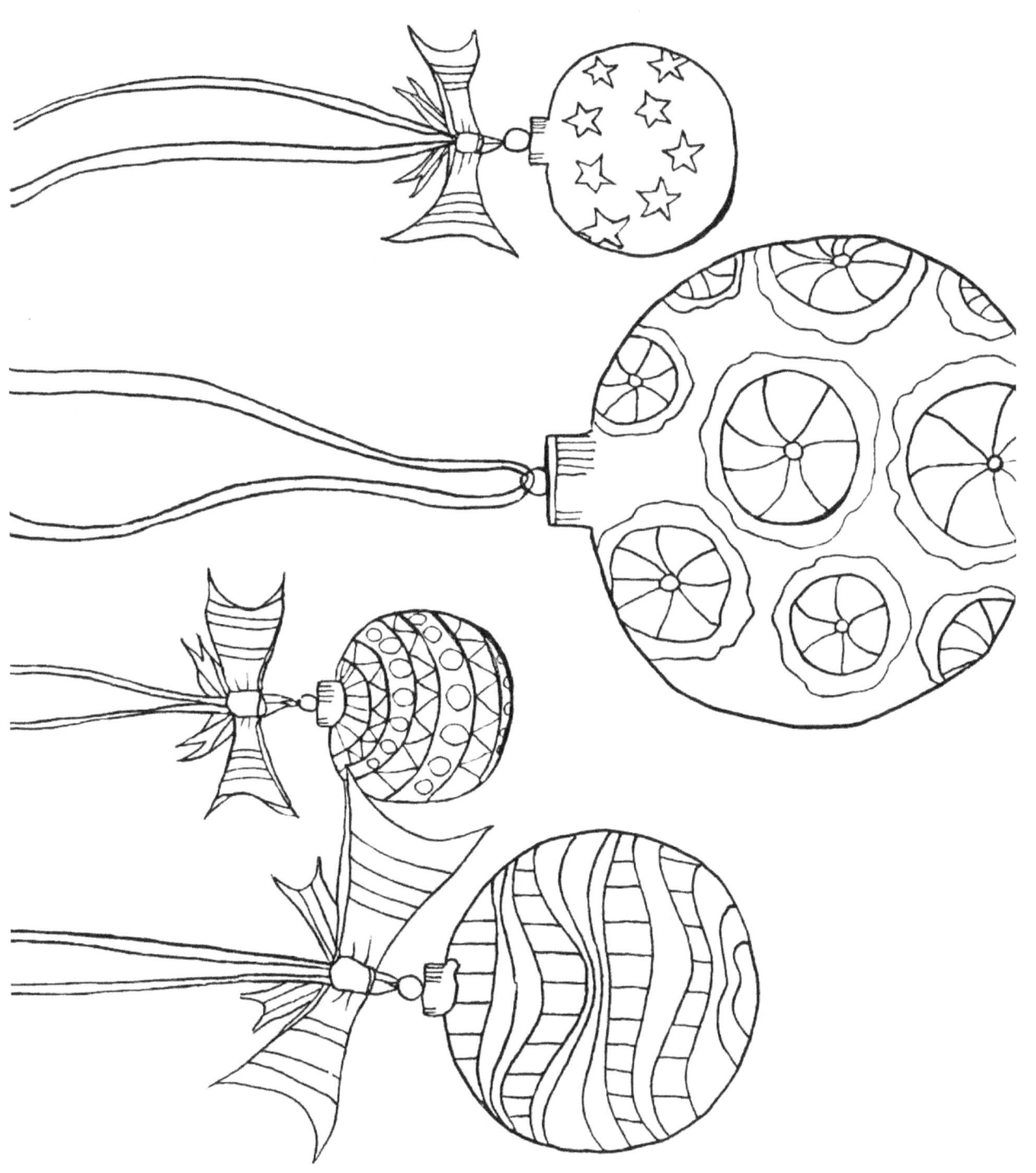

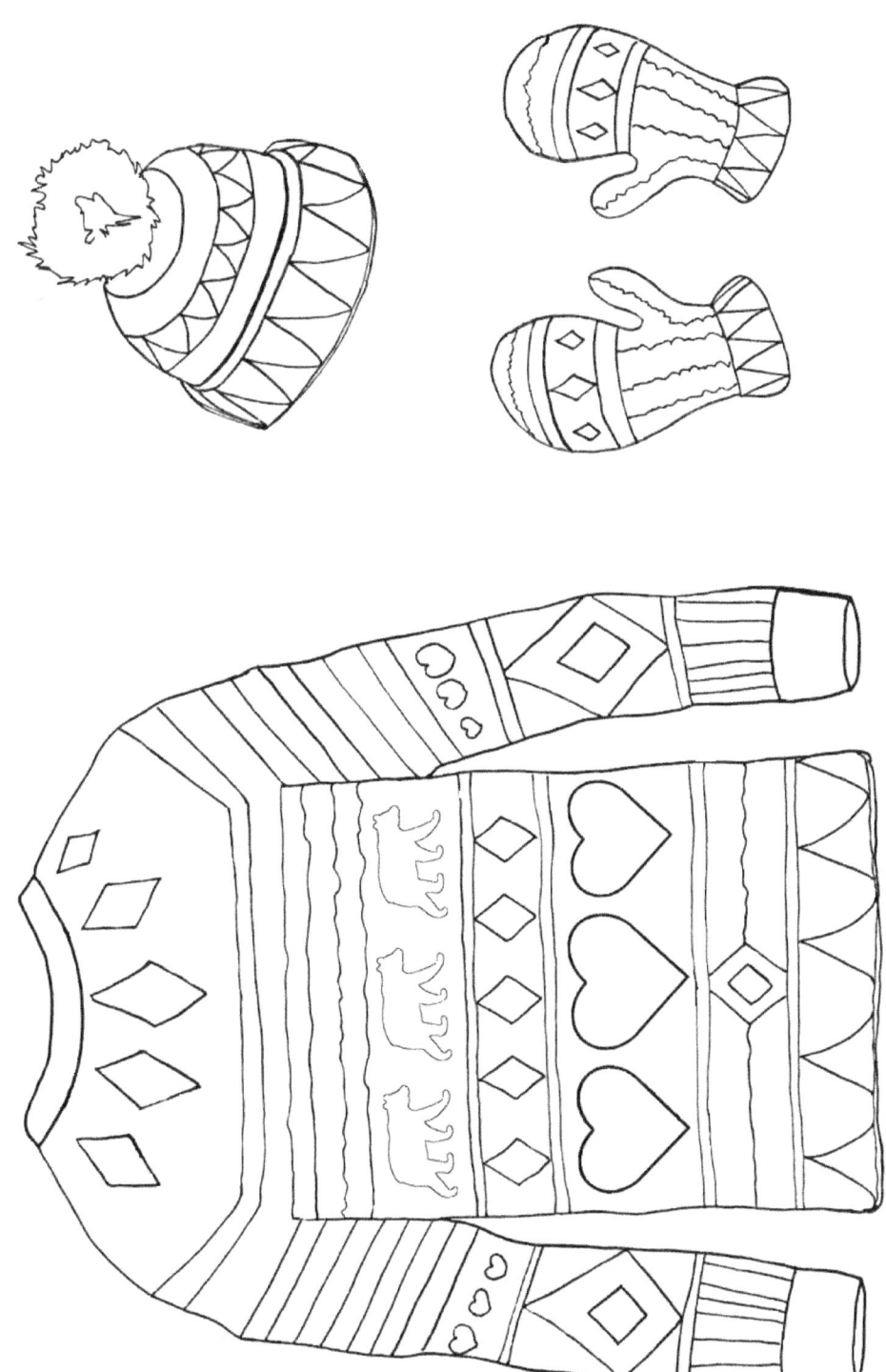

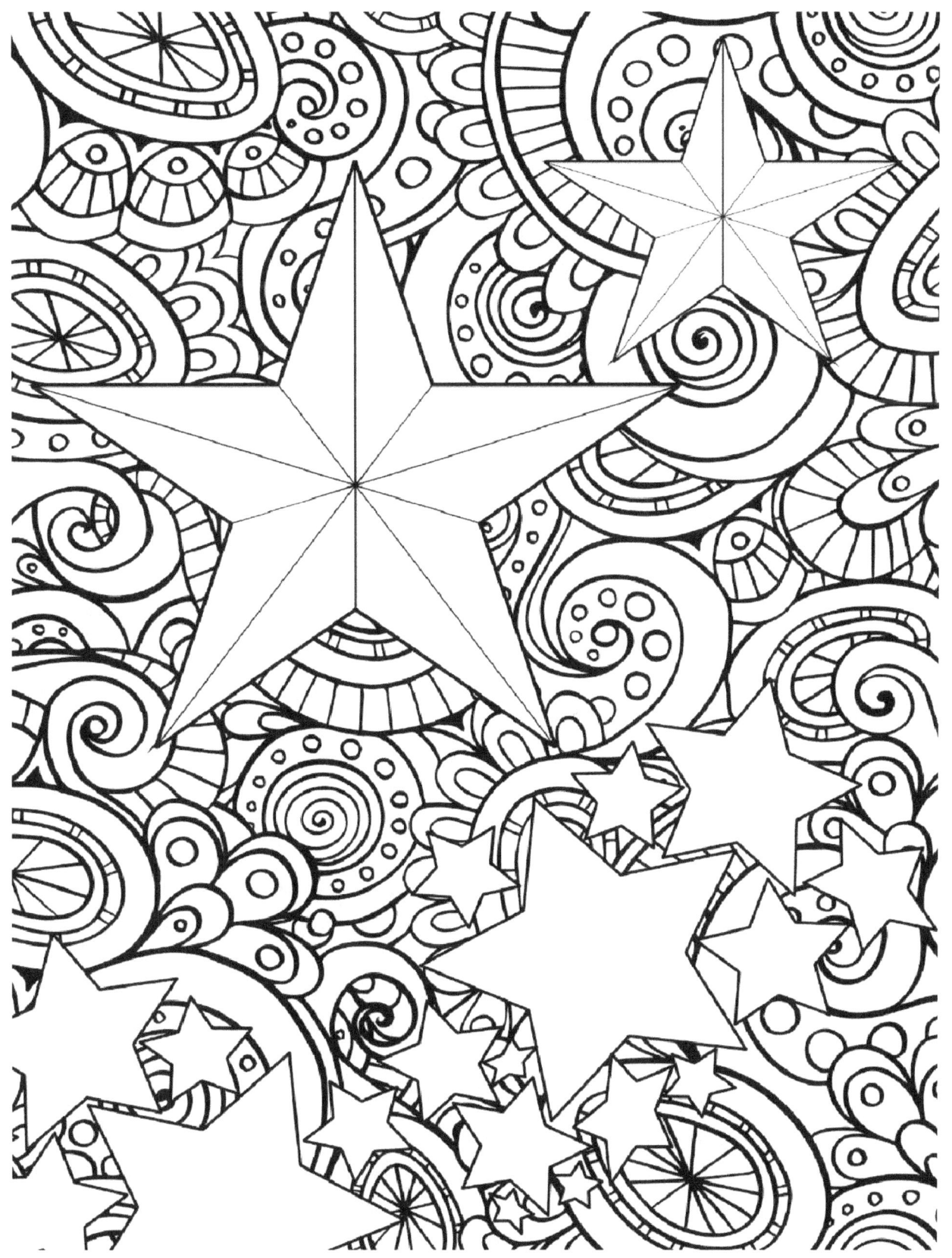

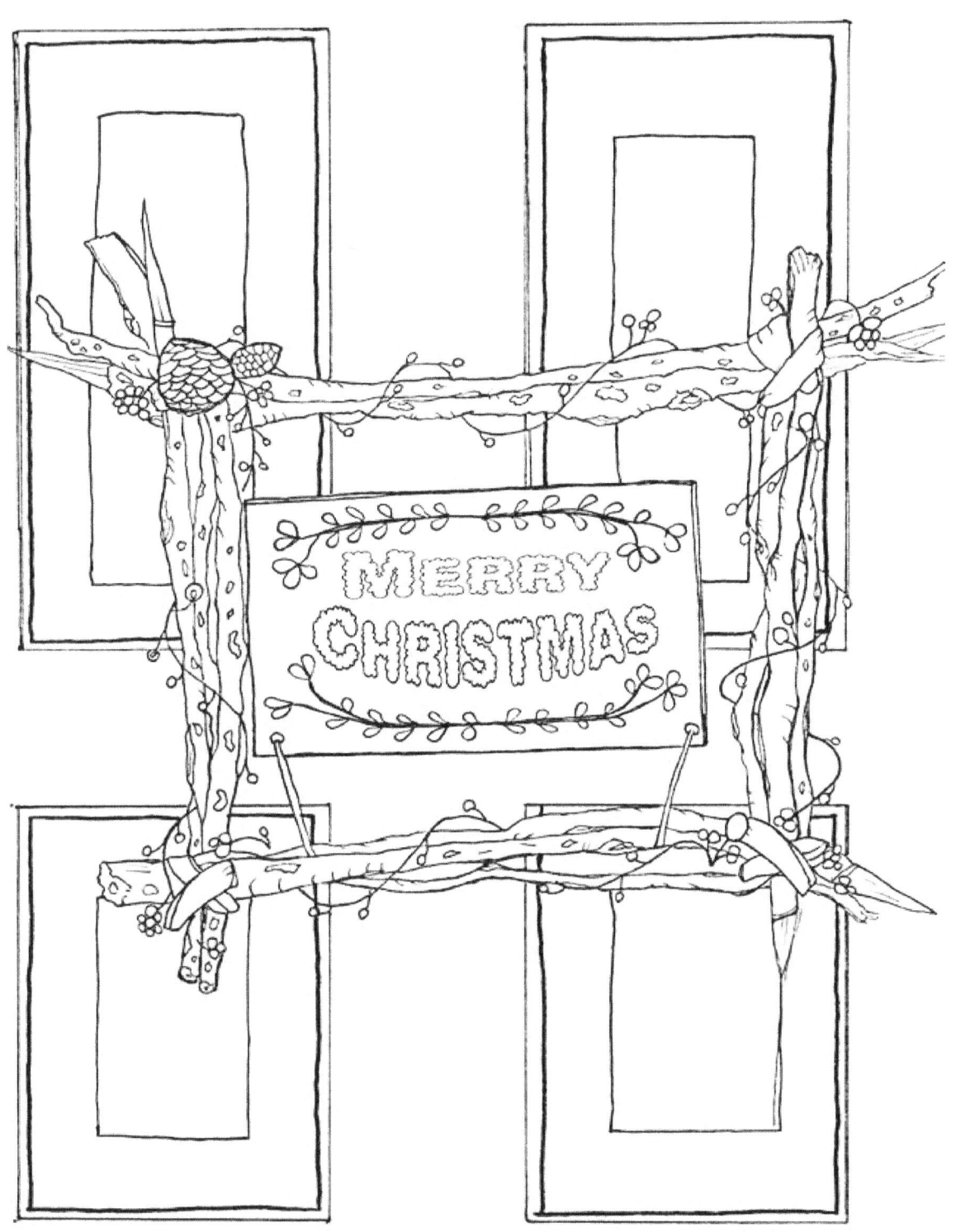

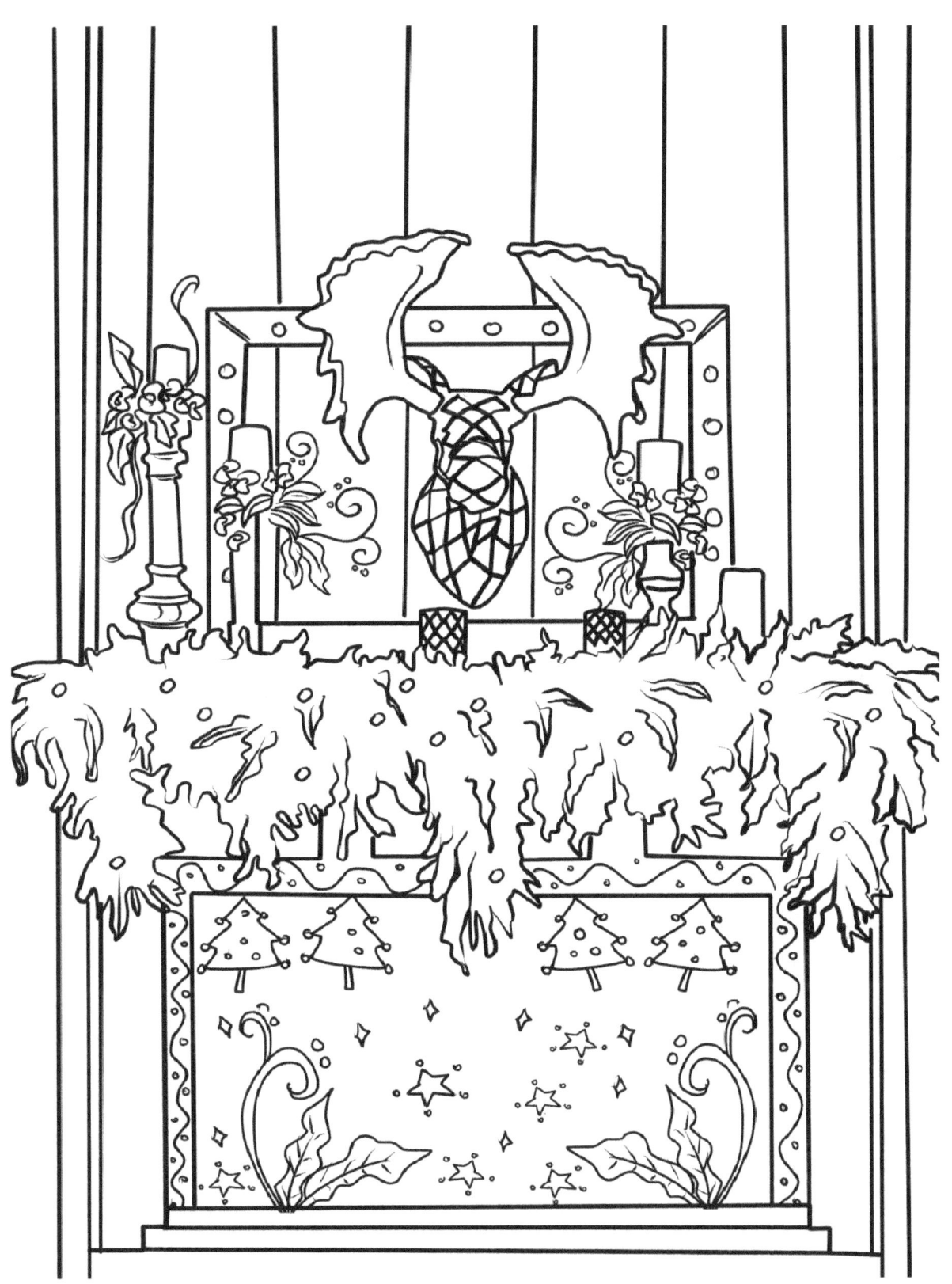

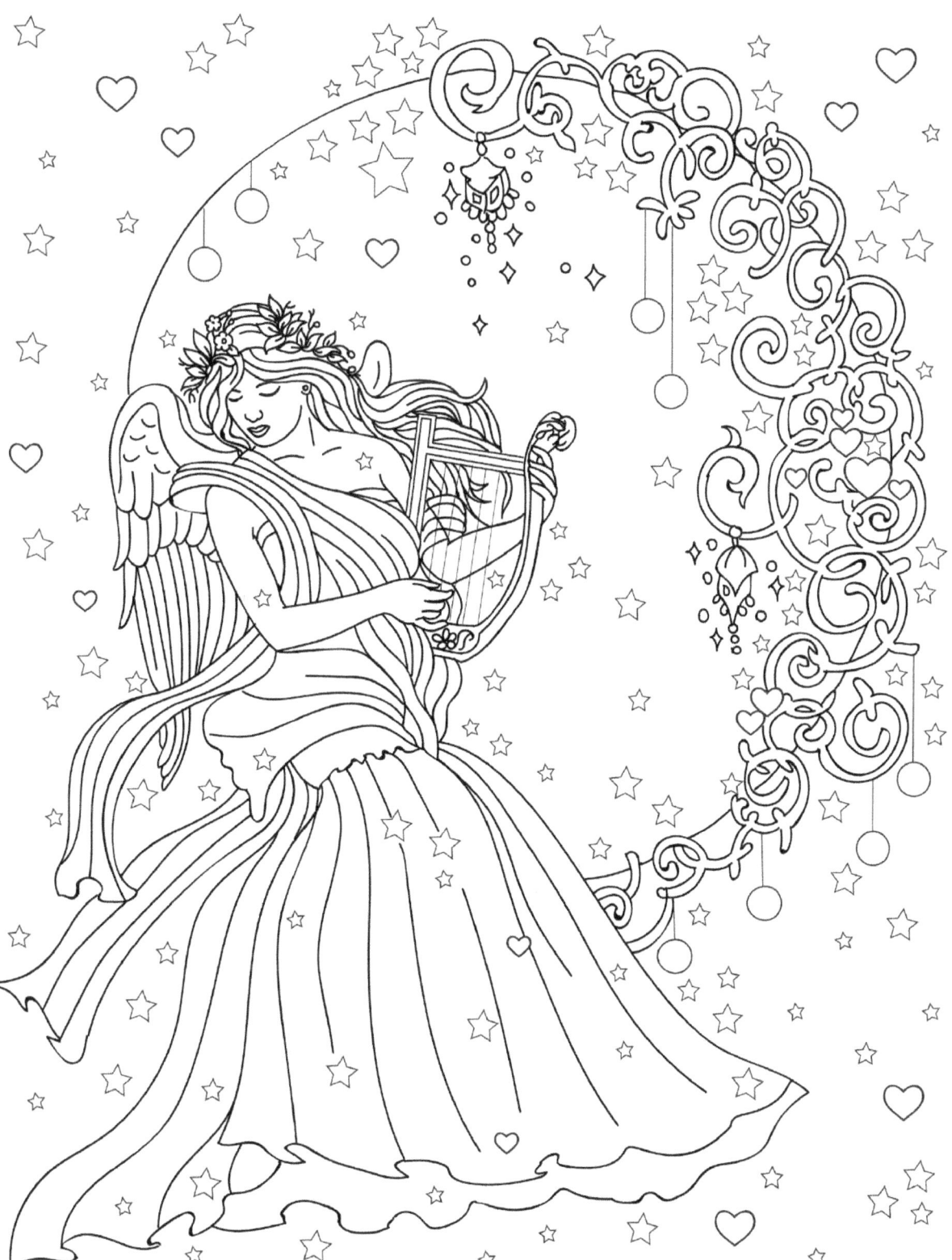

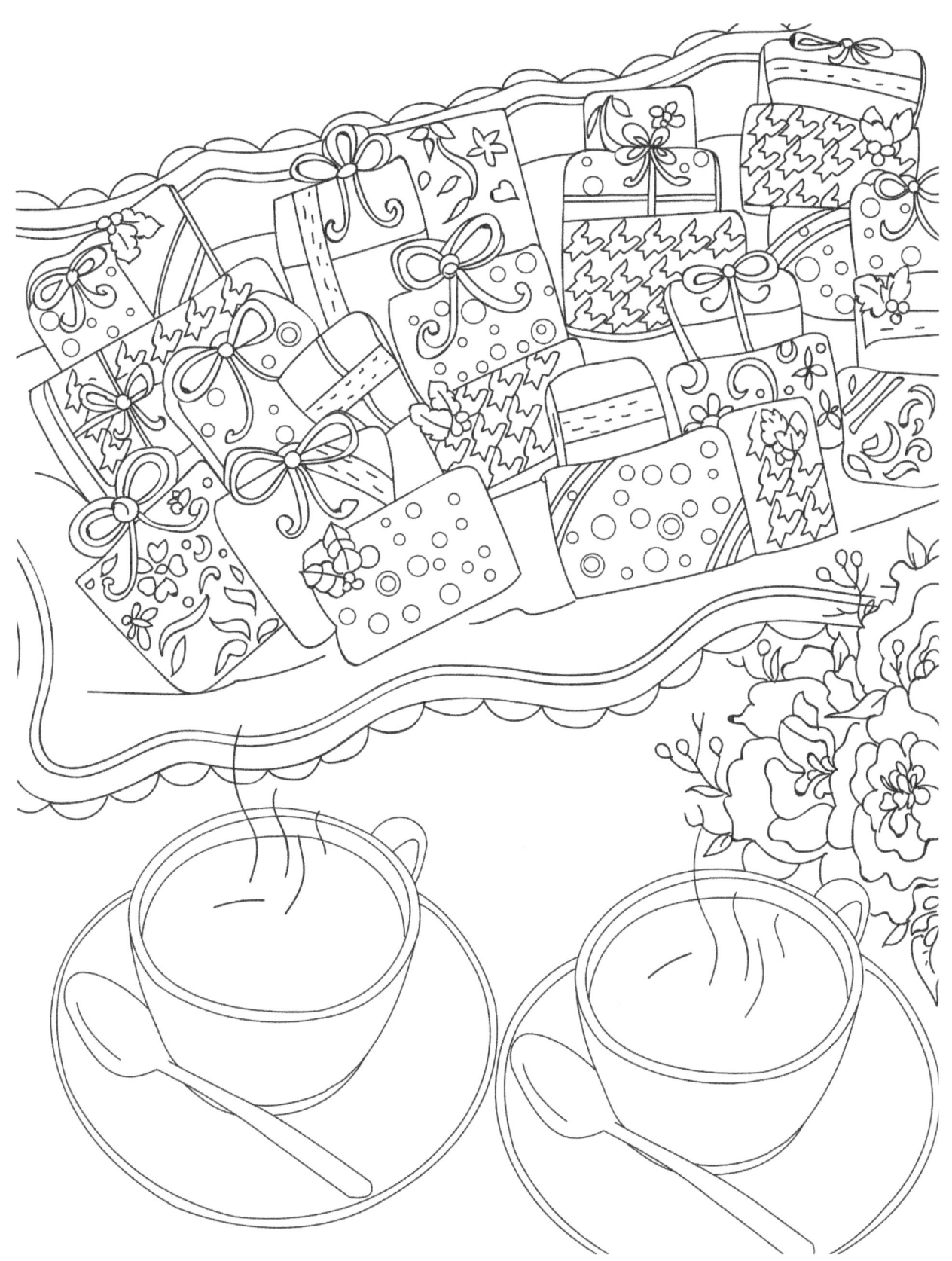

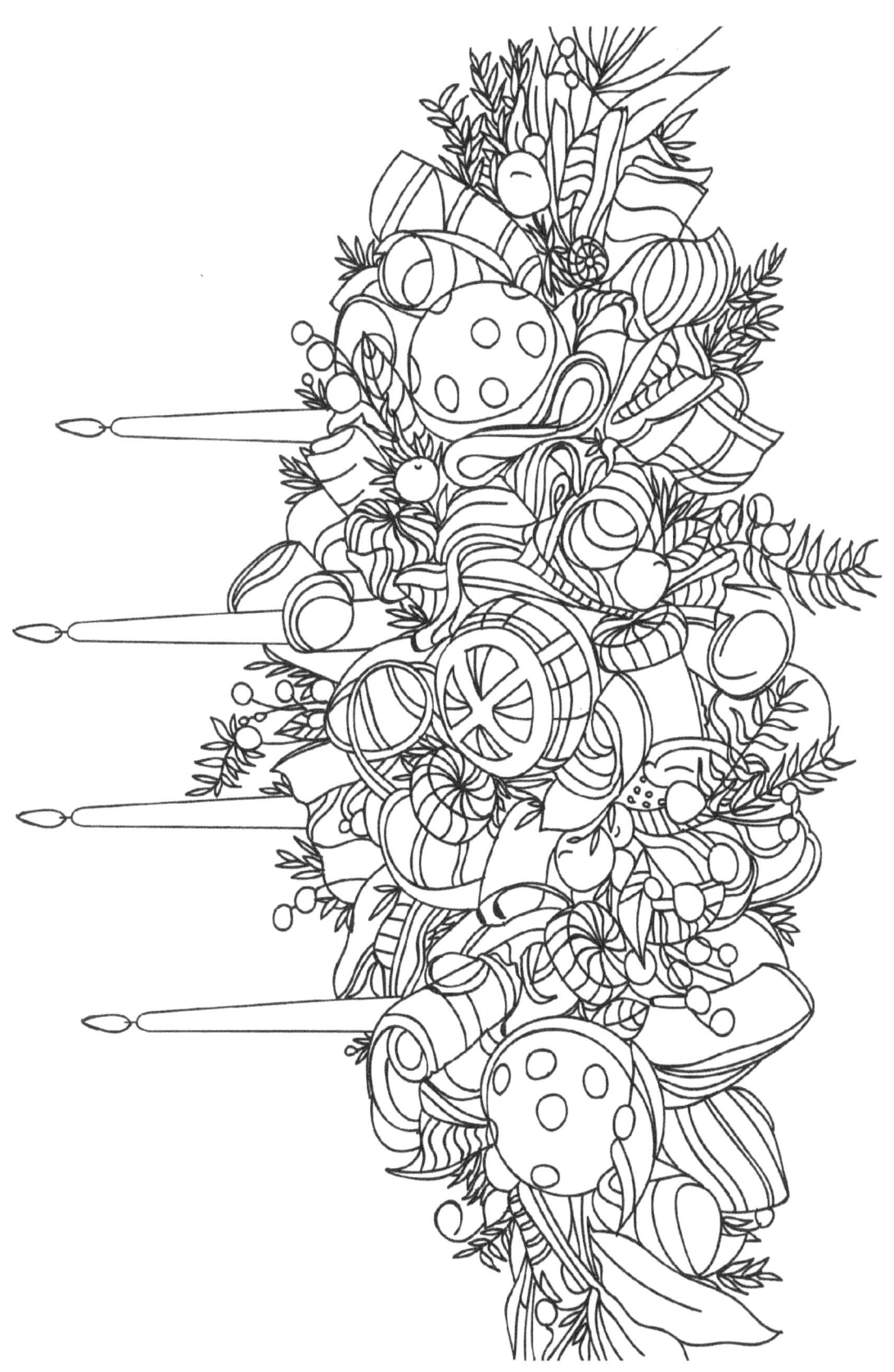

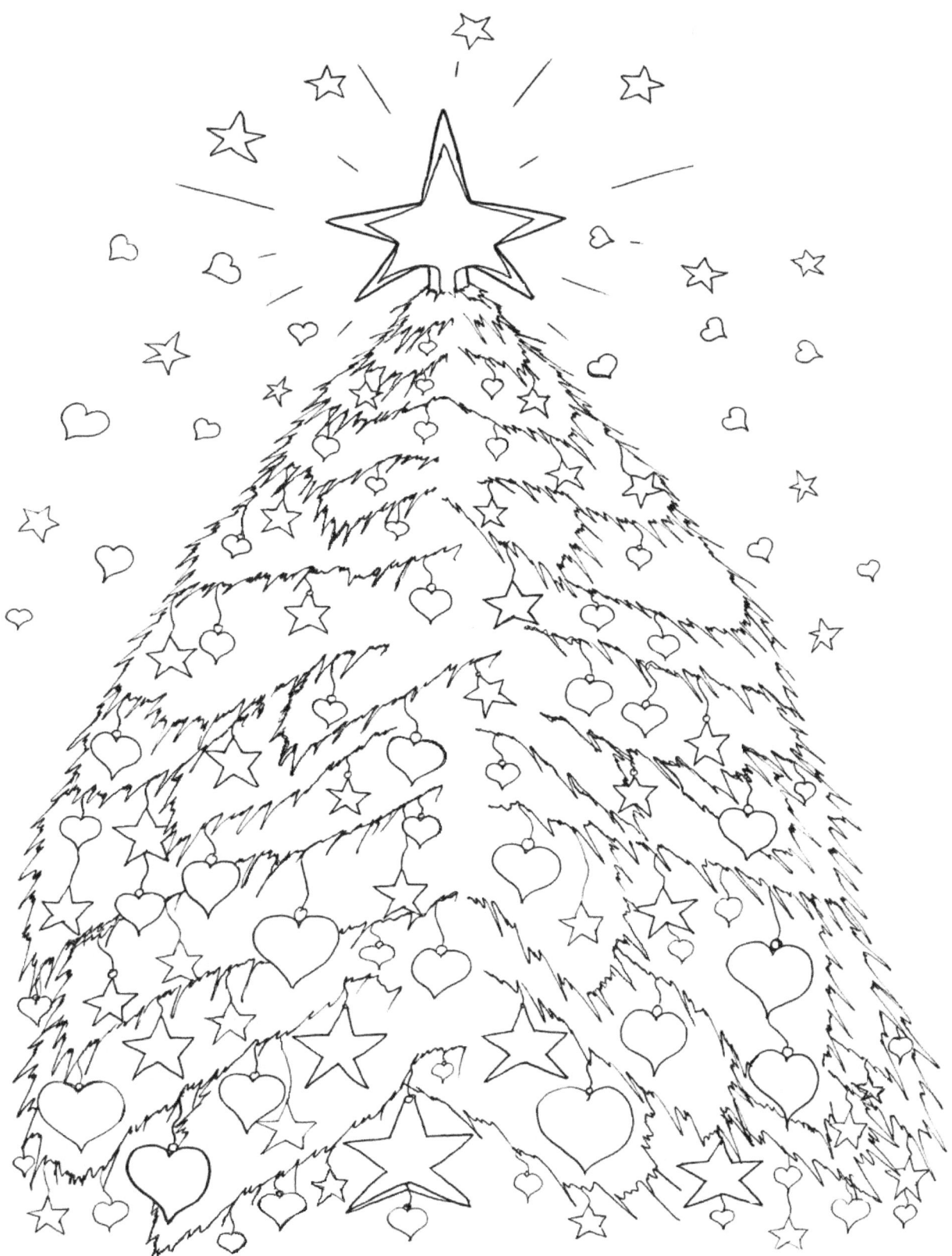

Thank You!

Thank you for purchasing the *Beautiful Christmas Coloring Book*. I so appreciate your patronage and hope that coloring in this book brought many sparkles and blessings to your preparation and celebration of this unique and beautiful Christmas holiday season!

If you enjoyed the *Beautiful Christmas Coloring Book*, then I would appreciate your honest review! Thanks so much already!

And if you are interested in learning more about my other products and publications, please visit:

http://www.adultcoloringbookseries.com

Merry Christmas!

www.ingramcontent.com/pod-product-compliance
Lightning Source LLC
Chambersburg PA
CBHW081752280526
45789CB00008B/2828

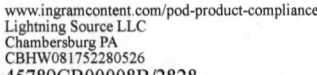